Disclaimer:

The information provided in this book is designed to provide helpful information on the subjects discussed. The publisher and author are not responsible for any specific health or allergy needs that may require medical supervision and are not liable for any damages or negative consequences from any treatment, action, application or preparation, to any person reading or following the information in this book.

Table of Contents

Introduction

Overview

Scrambled eggs with walnuts

Tasty Grilled Chicken

Crunchy Red Apple Butter

Almond Meal

Flat Belly Carrot Recipes

Ultimate Red Apple Meal

World Best Walnuts salad

Crunchy Spinach

Chicken Breast with Eggs

Mushroom Stir-fry with Delicious shrimp

Zero Belly Raisins Oat Meal

Vegetable Wrap-ups and Scrambled Eggs

Broccoli Vinaigrette

Flavorful Apple Stew and Autumn Chicken

Flat Belly Soup

Green Tea Smoothie with Berries

Black Cherry Delight

Exotic Chicken Salad

Sweet and Sour tomato salad

Healthy Greek Salad

Eggplant Tomato Salad

Half-Homemade Soup with Asparagus

Pork with Veggies

Salmon with Lemon and Dill

Chicken Parmigiana with Penne

Beef Stir-Fry Butternut Squash Soup

Jambalaya Blend with Veggies

Cod with Rosemary Polenta and Beans

Cookout for One

Oriental Garden Toss

Conclusion

Thank You

Introduction

Have ever thought of having a flat belly and still eat delicious meals? Well it will be a dream come true if you burn the excess fat in your tummy; with "The Belly Fat Burner: Ultimate Guideline to Lose Belly Fat Quick with 30 Delicious Recipes!" you will achieve your dreams of having an attractive, slim abs.

Having a flat belly is a paragon of good health and good shape. Everyday people seek to know the best workouts, products and recipes that would help them solve their problem of belly fat in order to look good. It is important to know losing belly fat isn't just about looking good; it is all about being healthy. Losing belly fat has so much lifesaving benefits that will help reduce the risk of several diseases such as diabetes, stroke and heart related problems. The negative thing about having belly fat; is that it is the most dangerous fat in the human body. Belly fat is located around your delicate organs like kidney, liver, heart and lungs. Belly fat is capable of destroying your health.

Belly fat is a stubborn body fat because it sticks to the stomach and hardly respond very well to workouts. Eating healthy and avoiding foods that are high in sugar and carbs will definitely help you burn and lose belly fat.

Having a flat, slim and sexy tummy seems to be a great deal and unachievable to most people who have little or no time for workouts, while some people have tried to lose belly fat with different types of workouts and foods which yielded no result. Now the good news I have for you is that there is a faster simple solution to lose belly fat and have a slim tummy. All you need to do is to thoroughly and thoughtfully follow the guidelines of this book, which will definitely help you have a flat tummy.

Personally I have used the guidelines I'm going to share in this book and have successfully gotten rid of my belly fat. And I'm so much excited about that. If these guidelines can work perfectly well for me, then it's the solution you have been looking for.

This book will teach you what you need to know about belly fat, why you still have belly fat and delicious recipes that will help you lose belly fat.

Having excess fat in the body is a great threat to physical fitness and more importantly to the health. That's the reason why people get concerned when they accumulate plenty fat in their body. Belly fat poses more threat than any other fat in the body because of where it is located. Belly fat has a lot of health risks and dangers.

Some health dangers of belly fat:

- Stroke
- Diabetes
- Cancer
- Heart related problems
- High blood pressure
- High cholesterol level

Belly fat generally can best be eliminated from the body in several ways like:

- Avoiding some bad habits and lifestyles like eating late t night, too much of junk foods and drinking too much soda and soft drinks which are very high in sugar.
- Eating healthy meals that are high in protein, fiber, low in carbohydrates and sugar is an effective way of reducing belly fat. Always eat fruits and vegetables like red apples, avocados, broccoli, watermelon, cucumber, cabbage, spinach.

- Always keep yourself hydrated by drinking plenty of clean water. And stop drinking sodas and other sugary drinks.
- Make sure you have enough sleep every night at least 7-8 hours, as this will help you get rid of belly fat.

Now there are a lot of things and you must avoid, if truly you want to lose belly fat. They are:

- Foods containing lots of white sugar
- Excessive alcohol
- Foods that are high in carbohydrates
- Sedentary lifestyle
- Plenty of white salt
- Artificial sweeteners
- Fried foods
- Foods that are high in saturated fat
- Stress
- Sodas and soft drinks
- Eating late at night
- Dairy products like cheese and butter

In addition to the recipes I will teach you in this book, you can also eat these simple foods, fruits and vegetables:

- Walnuts
- Flaxseeds
- Cinnamon

- Wild salmon

- Cherries

- Berries

- Black coffee

- Avocados

- Skinless turkey

- Red apples

- Watermelon

- Cucumber

- Leafy vegetables

- Green tea

- Banana

- Greek yogurt

- Tomatoes

- Mushrooms

- Almonds

Let's get started!

Scrambled eggs with walnuts

Serves 2

Ingredients:

3 eggs

½ cup chopped basil

1/3 cup chopped walnuts

Pepper

How you make it:

1. Whisk eggs in a bowl, then place in frying pan on medium heat, stirring continuously.
2. When eggs have almost cooked through, add the basil and continue cooking for another minute or until eggs is cooked through.
3. Add pepper to taste.
4. Remove from heat and stir in walnuts before serving.

Tasty Grilled Chicken

Serves 3-4

Ingredients:

4lb. Boneless, skinless chicken breast

2 teaspoon lime zest

¾ cup fresh lemon juice

¾ cup fresh lime juice

½ tablespoon granulated sugar

2 teaspoon lemon zest

2 teaspoon garlic, minced

¼ teaspoon cayenne pepper

¼ cup olive oil

How you make it:

1. In a small saucepan, whisk the lemon and lime zests and juices with the sugar, minced garlic and cayenne pepper.
2. Warm for about 5 minutes, until the sugar is dissolved. Whisk in the oil.
3. Remove from the stove and let the marinade cool.
4. Arrange the chicken breast in a large dish.
5. Try to set it up so the chicken is in a single layer. Prick the meat in several places with a fork and pour the marinade over the top.

6. Let the chicken marinate, covered and chilled for at least 3 hours, turning once. (You may opt to marinate the chicken overnight, if you prefer).

7. Using tongs, transfer the chicken to an oiled preheated grill.

8. Baste the chicken with the marinade and turn the meat at least 3 times while cooking, basting each time you turn.

9. Grill until chicken is cooked through.

Crunchy Red Apple Butter

Serves 4

Ingredients:

6 red apples

6 cups apple juice

1 cup sugar

½ teaspoon ground cloves spices

2 teaspoons cinnamon

1 teaspoon fresh lemon juice

How you make it:

1. Core and thinly slice apples into a large heavy saucepan.
2. Add apple juice until soft, about 30 minutes.
3. Pour red apples into a large sieve and press until all fruits passes through and leaves skin.
4. Discard skin. Repeat process until all apples are sieved.
5. Return pulp to the heavy sauce pan and boil gently, stirring frequently until thick.
6. Stir in sugar, spices and lemon juice. Cook , stirring over low heat for about one hour
7. Pour into sterilized ½ pint jars leaving ¼ inch headspace; adjust lids and process in a boiling water bath for 10 minutes after water comes to boil. You can successfully make half this recipe if desired.

Almond Meal

Serves 2

Ingredients:

2lbs. Asparagus

2 tablespoon olive oil

¾ cup slivered almonds, toasted

¼ teaspoon pepper

1 tablespoon lemon juice

How you make it:

1. Snap off tough ends of asparagus. Cook asparagus in boiling water to cover 3 minutes or until crisp- tender; drain.
2. Plunge asparagus into ice water to stop the cooking process; drain.
3. Add oil to large skillet over medium heat; add asparagus and sauté 3-5 minutes.
4. Toss asparagus with lemon juice and remaining ingredients.

Flat Belly Carrot Recipes

Serves 4

Ingredients:

6 med carrots, thinly sliced

6 teaspoon orange juice

½ teaspoon olive oil

¾ teaspoon ground cinnamon

1 teaspoon freshly ground black pepper

How you make it:

1. Place the carrots and orange juice in a medium saucepan.
2. Cover and cook over medium-low heat for 6minutes or until the carrots are tender crisp.
3. Add the oil, cinnamon and pepper. Cook for one minute stirring to coat.

Ultimate Red Apple Meal

Serving 3-4

Ingredients:

2 ¾ small red apples

1 cup coarsely grated carrots

½ cup vanilla nonfat Greek yogurt

5 cups green cabbage that is coarsely chopped

½ cup raisins

½ cup sun flower seeds (toasted, raw unsalted)

½ cup chopped fresh dill

5 cups red cabbage that is coarsely chopped

2 tablespoon apple cider vinegar

2 tablespoons olive oil

How you make it:

1. Combine red apples, carrots, raisins, sunflower seeds and cabbages in very large bowl.
2. To blend, whisk yogurt, olive oil, vinegar and dill in medium bowl.
3. To cabbage mixture add dressing and toss to distribute evenly.
4. Add pepper and salt to taste.

Tips: to make this easy for you, you can prepare this meal 3 hours ahead. After which you cover and refrigerate.

<h1 style="text-align:center">World Best Walnuts salad</h1>

Serves 2

Ingredients:

¼ cup olive oil

1 lb. watercress, finely chopped

½ cup cooked and finely diced chicken pieces

¼ cup walnuts, finely chopped

1 large garlic clove

¼ cup hazelnuts, finely chopped

½ teaspoon pepper

How you make it:

1. In a heavy 12-inch skillet, heat the olive oil.
2. Cut the garlic half lengthwise and add it to the oil. Cook for 2minutes, stirring constantly.
3. Remove the garlic and discard. Add all the nuts and cook for 5-6 minutes or until they are browned.
4. Add the chicken and pepper. Cook for 2-3minutes.
5. Dry watercress before adding it to oil.
6. Working fast, toss the watercress into the mixture in the pan, making sure it is well coated and barely heated through. If left for too long it loses some of its crispness.

7. Serve immediately.

Crunchy Spinach

Serves 1- 2

Ingredients:

2 eggs

½ teaspoon olive oil

2 cups fresh spinach

1 clove, garlic grated

How you make it:

1. Remove stems.
2. Wash the spinach thoroughly in warm salt water. Rinse.
3. Chop coarsely, until spinach wilts.
4. Beat in garlic and eggs. Heat olive oil, in medium saucepan.
5. Pour in egg mixture. Cook for about 2 minutes on each side, until egg is firm.
6. Serve.

<h1 style="text-align:center">Chicken Breast with Eggs</h1>

Serves 1-2

Ingredients:

2 boneless, skinless chicken breast, sliced into fingers

1 egg, beaten

½ teaspoon sea salt

½ teaspoon poultry seasoning

½ cup almond floor

1 teaspoon dry mustard powder

1/3 cup olive oil or coconut oil for frying.

How you make it:

1. Heat the oil in a large pan over medium heat.
2. Place the beaten egg in one bowl and the almond flour plus seasoning in another bowl.
3. Dip each chicken breast in egg, then in the almond flour mixture.
4. Cook the chicken in two batches until its golden on each side.

Mushroom Stir-fry with Delicious shrimp

Serving 4

Ingredients:

2 cups sliced mushrooms

1 teaspoon sesame oil

1 teaspoon olive oil

1 clove garlic, grated

½ teaspoon grated fresh ginger

1 cup okra

½ cup chopped green pepper

2 cups string beans

¼ teaspoon ground black pepper

2 cups cleaned cooked shrimps

How to make it:

1. Combine and stir- fry mushrooms, garlic, peppers, and ginger in sesame oil and olive oil until crisp-tender.
2. Meanwhile steam string beans and okra until crisp-tender.
3. Drain, and add peppers and mushrooms.
4. Stir in shrimp and pepper until just warmed.
5. Serve over a bed of lettuce.

Zero Belly Raisins Oat Meal

With this recipe you will get the chance to enjoy a tasty oat meal that is made in the traditional way.

Freshly baked, this meal will leave you incredibly full while helping you build muscles and burn belly fat.

Serves 2 bowls

Ingredients:

1 teaspoon vegetable oil

2 eggs, whites only

2 tablespoon of milk, skim

1/8 teaspoon of salt

½ cup of oats, Quick and Cooking variety

1 tablespoon of raisins

1/8 teaspoon of ground cinnamon

¼ teaspoon of baking powder

½ teaspoon of brown sugar

1 scoop of protein powder, vanilla or chocolate

How you make it:

1. Using a large mixing bowl, take your brown sugar and oil and whisk together until evenly combined.
2. Then slowly add in your oats, raisins, egg whites, baking powder, protein powder, skim milk and salt.
3. Top with your brown sugar and ground cinnamon.
4. Cover with some plastic wrap and place into your refrigerator. Let it sit overnight.
5. The next day take out your oat meal and place into greased baking dish.
6. Preheat your oven to 350 degrees and then bake your oatmeal for about 35minutes or until oatmeal is firm.
7. Remove from heat and serve.

<h1 align="center">Vegetable Wrap-ups and Scrambled Eggs</h1>

Serving 8

Ingredients:

1 teaspoon olive oil

2 scallions, chopped

1 tablespoon onion chopped

1 green pepper, chopped

2 cups sliced mushrooms

8 romaine lettuce leaves

½ teaspoon ground black pepper

1 tablespoon taco seasoning mix, dry

8 eggs (4 egg whites)

¾ cup shredded cheddar cheese

How you make it:

1. Coat a large skillet with olive oil. Sauté green pepper, onion and mushroom until tender.
2. Transfer vegetable to small bowl. Stir in scallions. Set aside.
3. On serving plates, sprinkle lettuce evenly with cheese.
4. Beat together eggs and egg whites. Stirring often until just firm and moist, in the same skillet cook eggs.

5. Divide eggs among lettuce leaves.

6. Divide vegetable mixture over eggs.

7. If necessary, roll up the lettuce leaves and secure them with toothpicks.

8. Serve immediately.

Broccoli Vinaigrette

Serves 6

Ingredients: 2 tablespoon white vinegar

½ pound fresh broccoli

½ teaspoon dry mustard

1 teaspoon olive oil

¼ teaspoon salt

¼ teaspoon ground black pepper

How you make it:

1. Trim the broccoli leaves and lower stems, after you have washed it.
2. Cut broccoli into spears.
3. Steam until crisp-tender, for about 5 minutes. Drain.
4. Combine mustard, vinegar, pepper, oil and salt.
5. Drizzle over broccoli.
6. Serve immediately.
7. Also good chilled, as cold leftovers.

Flavorful Apple Stew and Autumn Chicken

Serves 4

Ingredients:

3 carrots, peeled, sliced

1 chicken, cut in parts

¼ cup apple cider vinegar

½ teaspoon nutmeg

6 red apples, peeled, sliced

6 whole cloves

1 cup shredded cabbage

½ teaspoon salt

¼ teaspoon pepper

2 teaspoons Dijon mustard

1 cup apple sauce

¾ cup low sodium chicken broth, warm

How you make it:

1. Heat large Dutch oven over medium high temperature, after spraying vegetable cooking spray.
2. Add chicken turning to brown on all sides, and cook for about 10miutes.
3. Sprinkle with nutmeg, pepper and salt.

4. Spread mustard over chicken pieces, and warm broth, cloves, carrots and vinegar. Bring to boil.

5. Reduce heat to low, cover and cook for 15minutes.

6. Add apples and cook for about 5minutes.

7. Add cabbage, stirring into liquid. Cook covered until fork can be inserted in chicken with ease, cook for about 10minutes more.

8. With slotted spoon, remove vegetables and chicken to warm serving bowl and keep warm.

9. Stir applesauce into liquid, boil on high temperature for about 5 minutes and pour over chicken and vegetables.

10. Serve with brown rice, if desired.

Flat Belly Soup

Serves 8

Ingredients:

2 quarts homemade chicken broth

1 pound spinach, thoroughly washed

4 eggs

¼ cup fresh basil leaves

¼ cup fresh parsley

2 tablespoons lemon juice

½ cup freshly grated parmesan cheese

½ teaspoon ground black pepper

How to make it:

1. Boil chicken broth in a large pan.
2. Remove stems from spinach.
3. Tear each leave in quarters.
4. Rinse and set aside.
5. Beat together parsley, basil, lemon juice, eggs, parmesan and pepper.
6. Set aside. 5 minutes before serving and working quickly, stir spinach into broth.
7. Cook for about a minute.

8. Using wire whisk, stir egg mixture into the broth, adding the eggs gradually so they don't clump.

9. This should be wispy looking.

10. Continue to whisk for about 2minutes until egg is cooked through.

11. Serve immediately.

<h1 style="text-align:center">Green Tea Smoothie with Berries</h1>

Serves 1

Ingredients:

¾ cup of fortified vanilla soy milk

½ medium sized banana

½ cup of frozen blueberries

2 teaspoon of honey

1 Green tea bag

½ glass of water

How you make it:

1. Place the water in a small bowl and heat in the microwave until it is steaming hot. Add the Green tea bag and let it brew for 3minutes. After you remove the bag, add the honey and stir until it sets.
2. Take out your blender and blend the milk, banana and berries.
3. Add the tea which you made in step 1 to the mixture which you blended in step 2. Blend all of the ingredients once again. If needed, add a bit more water to the mixture.
4. Pour the delicious smoothie out and serve in a tall glass.

Black Cherry Delight

Serves1

Ingredients:

1 cup almond milk

3 ice cubes

1 tablespoon flaxseed

½ cup frozen black cherries

1 tablespoon cacao

How you make it:

1. Mix the milk and frozen cherries in a blender and then add the rest.
2. Blend until smooth and creamy.
3. Serve in a tall glass.

Note: you can add frozen blueberries too, you would definitely love it!

Exotic Chicken Salad

Serves 8

Ingredients:

1 Honeydew melon

6cups cubed, cooked chicken meat

2 cups chopped celery

2 cups seedless grapes

1 (8ounce) can sliced, water chestnuts

½ cup sour cream

½ cup plain yogurt

½ teaspoon curry powder

Salt and pepper to taste

How to make it:

1. Wash the melon.
2. Cut melon into half, and remove seeds.
3. Cut melon into bite-size pieces.
4. Add chicken, celery, grapes and water chestnuts.
5. Whisk together sour cream, yogurt and curry powder in a small bowl.
6. Gently stir into salad.
7. Season with pepper and salt to taste.
8. Serve.

Sweet and Sour tomato salad

Serves 3

Ingredients:

7 Tomatoes

1 Small yellow onion

½ cup distilled white vinegar

½ cup vegetable oil

Salt and pepper to taste

How to make it:

1. Wash the tomatoes and onion.
2. Slice the tomatoes thinly.
3. Cut the onion into half, then thinly slice into half circles.
4. In a large bowl, combine tomatoes, onion, vinegar, oil, salt and pepper.
5. Serve at room temperature.

Healthy Greek Salad

Serves 3

Ingredients:

3 Large ripe tomatoes, chopped

2 cucumbers, peeled and chopped

1 Small red onion chopped

¼ cup olive oil

4 teaspoons lemon juice

½ teaspoon oregano

Salt and pepper to taste

1 cup crumbled feta cheese

6 Black Greek olives, pitted and sliced

How to make it:

1. Wash tomatoes, cucumber and onion.
2. Combine tomatoes, cucumber and onion in a bowl.
3. Sprinkle with oil, lemon juice, oregano.
4. Add salt and pepper to taste.
5. Sprinkle feta cheese and olives over salad.
6. Serve.

Eggplant Tomato Salad

Serves 2-3

Ingredients:

1 Green bell pepper

1 Large red bell pepper

7 Tomatoes

1 Eggplant

4 Cloves crushed garlic

¼ cup extra virgin oil

2 Tablespoons tomato paste

½ teaspoon salt

½ teaspoon ground black pepper

½ teaspoon cayenne pepper

How to make it:

1. Roast pepper until skin turns black.
2. Cool in a plastic bag.
3. Remove burnt skin and rinse well.
4. Boil tomatoes for 1 minute and cool in ice water.
5. Peel and chop tomatoes.
6. Cut the eggplant into small strips and sauté in oil for about 6-8 minutes.
7. Once the eggplant is soft add garlic.
8. Open the peppers and remove seeds.
9. Cut pepper into small strips and add to eggplant.

10. Add tomatoes to eggplant mixture.

11. Add tomatoes paste, salt, pepper and cayenne.

12. Bring to boil, reduce heat and simmer for 30 minutes.

13. Let the salad cool before serving.

Half-Homemade Soup with Asparagus

Serves 4

Ingredients:

4 Oz boneless, skinless chicken breast

2 tablespoons quinoa

1 cup Amy's organic chunky vegetable soup

1 cup chopped kale

10 small Asparagus spears

2 teaspoon soy sauce

¼ teaspoon grated fresh ginger

How to make it:

1. Wash chicken breast.
2. Bake chicken at 350 degrees for 25 minutes.
3. Shred the chicken with a fork.
4. Combine soup, quinoa, and kale in a saucepan.
5. Boil and simmer for 15 minutes until quinoa is done.
6. Add chicken.
7. Steam asparagus, then toss with soy sauce and ginger.
8. Serve asparagus on the side.

Pork with Veggies

Serves 2-3

Ingredients:

1 Pork tenderloin (4oz)

1 cup steamed beans

2 Tablespoons sliced almonds

1 baked sweet potato

How to make it:

1.   Season pork with salt and pepper.

2.   Sear in an ovenproof skillet coated with cooking spray.

3.   Transfer to a 450 degrees oven for 15 minutes.

4.   Slice and serve with green beans topped with almonds and sweet potato.

Salmon with Lemon and Dill

Serves 4

Ingredients:

5 oz wild Atlantic salmon

1 tablespoon lemon juice

1teaspoon dill

2/3 cup parsnips

½ cup chopped broccoli, steamed

How to make it:

1.   Sprinkle salmon with lemon juice and dill.

2.   Bake for 15 minutes at 250 degrees.

3.   Serve.

Chicken Parmigiana with Penne

Serves 3

Ingredients:

4 oz grilled chicken, diced

½ cup tomato sauce

1 cup spinach

½ cup whole- wheat penne

½ tablespoon grated Parmesan

How to make it:

1.   Sauté spinach in one teaspoon olive oil.

2.   Toss with chicken, penne and tomato sauce.

3.   Top with parmesan.

4.   Serve.

Beef Stir-Fry Butternut Squash Soup

Serves 3

Ingredients:

3 oz steak tenderloin fillet, sliced thin

½ cup sliced shiitake mushrooms

½ onion, sliced

1/3 cup cooked bulgur

Butternut squash soup

How to make it:

1.   Stir-fry beef, onion and mushrooms.

2.   Serve over bulgur.

Jambalaya Blend with Veggies

Serves 2-3

Ingredients:

1 veggie burger

½ cup cooked brown rice

2 tablespoons corn

2 tablespoons salsa

½ cup chopped red, green or yellow bell peppers

¾ cup diced squash

¾ cup diced zucchini

¼ cup chopped red onion

1 teaspoon olive oil

Salt to taste

How to make it:

1.   Cook burger in a pan sprayed with cooking spray.

2.   Chop burger and combine with rice, corn and salsa.

3.   Toss veggies with oil and salt.

4.   Then roast for 15-20 minutes.

5.   Serve on the side.

Cod with Rosemary Polenta and Beans

Serves 2

Ingredients:

3 oz cod

1 teaspoon chopped fresh parsley

Dash of salt

Dash of pepper

¼ cup dry polenta

½ cup 1 percent milk

1 tablespoon pine nuts

½ teaspoon rosemary

½ cup cooked green beans

How to make:

1.	Season cod with parsley, salt and pepper.

2.	Then steam for 8 minutes.

3.	Cook polenta with milk.

4.	Then top with pine nuts and rosemary.

5.	Serve with green beans.

Serving 2

Ingredients:

1 organic beef hot dog

½ cup organic baked beans

1 whole-wheat hot dog bun

½ tablespoon whole grain mustard

½ tablespoon sweet relish

1 cup sliced honeydew melon

How to make it:

1.	Cook hot dog.

2.	Heat baked beans in a saucepan.

3.	Serve hot dog in the bun.

4.	Top with mustard and relish.

5.	Add beans and melon on the side.

Oriental Garden Toss

Serves 6

Ingredients:

1/3 cup thinly sliced green onions

1 tablespoon reduced-sodium soy sauce

3 tablespoons water

½ teaspoon roasted sesame oil

3 packets EQUAL sweetener

¼ teaspoon garlic powder

1/8 teaspoon crushed red pepper flakes

1 package (3 oz) low-fat ramen noodles soup

2 cups fresh peas pod, halved crosswise

1 cup fresh bean sprouts

 1 cup sliced fresh mushrooms

1 can (8 3/4 oz) baby corn, drained and halved crosswise

1 red bell pepper, cut into bit-size strips

3 cups shredded Chinese cabbage

How to make it:

1.   Combine green onions, soy sauce, water, sesame oil, equal, garlic powder and red pepper flakes in screw-top jar, set aside.

2.   Breakup ramen noodles (discard seasoning packet).

3.   Combine with pea pods in large bowl.

4.   Pour boiling water over mixture to cover.

5.   Let stand one minute drain.

6.   Combine noodles, pea pods, bean sprouts, mushrooms, baby corn and bell pepper in a large bowl.

7.   Shake dressing and add to noodle mixture, toss to coat.

8.   Cover and chill 2-24 hours.

9.   Just before serving add shredded cabbage, toss to combine.

Conclusion

I want to encourage you to take the guidelines of this book serious, to commit to something, because when you commit to something and you actually do it and stick with it, it builds up the habit and real power. When was the last time you had a goal you actually set up and feel good about it? I want you to get this in your mind that we always need new goals in life.

The coolest thing about this is that if you do it with somebody and you encourage them to follow the guidelines of this book like a friend, family, relative or virtual community. It would help you greatly to stick to your goals and stay committed.

The guidelines of this book have helped transformed lives, with lots of testimonies. Always be positive in following this book. Take a massive action in your life today, because your transformation and losing belly fat would affect positive changes on you, make you happy and everyone around you.

If you follow religiously to my 10 Day Smoothies Recipes https://www.amazon.com/dp/B06X6BTSGQ and the delicious recipes outlined in this book. You will definitely see great results in your body and health in no distant time, because it is proven to work.

If you enjoyed the guidelines and recipes in this book, please take the time to share your thoughts and post a positive review with 5star rating on Amazon, it would encourage me and make me serve you better. It would be greatly appreciated.

9 781978 252073